A GUIDE TO HAWAIIAN MASSAGE

The Hawaiian Massage Experience: Uncovering The Secrets Of Lomi Lomi

ABRAM ROBIN

Contents

CHAPTER ONE
Hawaiian Massage: An Overview

Hawaiian massage is a healing art that has been practiced on the islands of Hawaii for generations.

This ancient Polynesian technique, also called Lomi Lomi massage, has been passed down from generation to generation and is revered for its comprehensive focus on wellness.

Hawaiian massage is more than just a set of physical strokes; it is an entire mind, body, and spirit ritual with the goal of reestablishing the balance and harmony that had been lost. It is a type of bodywork that involves the therapist applying pressure and kneading the muscles with rhythmic motions, long flowing strokes, and the use of their hands, forearms, and elbows. Relaxing music and fragrant oils are common accompaniments to the massage as the receiver lies face up on a massage table.

Hawaiian massage is distinctive in that it is informed by a philosophy that considers the mind, emotions, and spirit to be an integral part of the body.

It is considered that optimum health and well-being can be attained when these factors are in harmony with one another. By easing muscular tension and opening up the body's energy channels, Hawaiian massage can help people feel better on many levels.

Hawaiian massage is well-known for more than just its general revitalizing and calming effects; it is also effective at relieving chronic pain, joint stiffness, and circulation disorders. It is a flexible and adaptable method of bodywork since it can be tailored to the specific requirements of each client.

In addition to its therapeutic benefits, a traditional Hawaiian massage is a spiritual and cultural journey into the heart of the Hawaiian people. Its genuineness and originality are enhanced by the inclusion of prayers, chants, and other traditional traditions.

Hawaiian massage can be a life-changing experience for anybody looking to unwind, reduce stress, or strengthen the bond between body and soul. Relax into the calming beats of this ancient art form and feel the aloha spirit of Hawaii wash over you. Mahalo!

Lomi Lomi's Philosophical Underpinnings

Lomi Lomi, commonly known as Hawaiian massage, takes a more comprehensive view of health and wellness than its physical practices alone. The guiding ideas and philosophy of Lomi Lomi are as follows:

• Lomi Lomi's foundation is the idea that people and the natural world around them are inextricably linked. To help their patients feel more at one with nature, practitioners frequently use sounds and images of water, ocean waves, and animal movements in their treatments.

• Lomi Lomi recognizes the interconnectedness of the mind, body, and spirit, and treats the whole person rather than just the parts. Realizing that disruptions in one area can have ripple effects throughout the whole, it seeks to bring equilibrium and harmony to all aspects of existence. Lomi Lomi practitioners think that the best way to heal is to address both the body's physical strain and the mind's emotional stress.

•The spirit of aloha refers to the importance of love, compassion, and connection in Hawaiian society. Those that practice Lomi Lomi do so with a pure desire to help those receiving it feel safe and cared for as they heal and refresh.

• Lomi Lomi is often compared to a dance of the hands due to its fluid motions and intuitive touch. The practitioner's intuition and the recipient's body connection inform their movements, which flow and have a natural rhythm. The result is a profound sense of letting go, relaxation, and surrender for the recipient.

• Huna Philosophy: Huna is a traditional Hawaiian philosophy that informs Lomi Lomi by emphasizing the unity of body, mind, and spirit. Huna says that true healing takes place when all factors are in harmony. Huna teachings and practices, like energy clearing, intention setting, and connecting to higher awareness, may be incorporated into Lomi Lomi sessions.

• Lomi Lomi is a form of Polynesian healing art with strong historical and cultural roots in Hawaii. Lomi Lomi sessions may include cultural rituals including prayers, chants, and ceremonies to pay homage to the tradition's ancestry and ancestors. The experience of Lomi Lomi is richer and more genuine because of this respect for tradition.

Overall, the beliefs and philosophy of Lomi Lomi reflect a holistic approach to healing, with an accent on the connectivity of body, mind, and spirit, the strength of intuition and flow, and a profound reverence for nature, tradition, and the aloha spirit. It is a rare and revered kind of massage that goes beyond the skin deep to foster whole-person health and wholeness via the power of touch.

CHAPTER TWO
Hawaiian Massage In Its Historical And Cultural Context

Hawaiian massage, also known as Lomi Lomi, has a rich cultural history that is connected with the traditions of the Hawaiian people.

The healing art of Lomi Lomi has been passed down through the generations from ancient Polynesia as a reflection of Hawaiian culture's spirituality, heritage, and value.

Traditionally, kahunas, the ancient Hawaiian society's spiritual leaders and healers, performed Lomi Lomi. They were respected members of society who looked out for the emotional, intellectual, and spiritual well of their fellow citizens.

Lomi Lomi was revered because it was thought to address not just the body but also the mind, spirit, and soul of its recipient.

Lomi Lomi is an integral part of Hawaiian culture because it exemplifies the affinity that Hawaiians have with the earth, the sea, and all things natural. The Hawaiian people place a premium on preserving natural resources and a harmonious relationship with the natural world.

The Hawaiians' strong respect for nature is shown in Lomi Lomi's incorporation of natural aspects like flowing water, ocean waves, and the movements of animals.

The aloha spirit, which is central to Hawaiian beliefs, is also present in

Lomi Lomi. It is considered that aloha is the very essence of existence, standing for love, compassion, and connection.

Practitioners of Lomi Lomi do their work with an open heart and a caring goal, fostering a relaxing and healing environment for the client.

Huna is a traditional Hawaiian philosophy that emphasizes the unity of body, mind, and spirit, and its teachings are embedded in Lomi Lomi. Huna says that true healing takes place when all factors are in harmony.

Huna methods, such as energy clearing, intention setting, and connecting to higher awareness, may be incorporated into Lomi Lomi sessions.

The Hawaiian people and others who have been trained in Lomi Lomi from other countries continue to practice and revere Lomi Lomi as a sacred healing art. Bodywork in the Hawaiian tradition is more than simply a massage; it is an immersion in the culture, history, and spirituality of the Hawaiian people.

Lomi Lomi's Foundational Moves And Strokes

Hawaiian massage, also known as Lomi Lomi, is characterized by fluid, rhythmic motions that involve the whole body, not just the hands. Lomi Lomi's strokes and techniques aim to alleviate stress, remove muscle tightness, and realign the whole person. Some of the most fundamental Lomi Lomi strokes and methods are as follows:

• Lomi Lomi is characterized by its use of long, sweeping strokes. Practitioners make fluid, undulating motions with their hands, forearms, and sometimes elbows, like the ebb and flow of ocean waves, all over the body. By using long, smooth strokes, the therapist can reduce muscle tension and induce a state of deep calm and surrender in the recipient.

• Lomi Lomi is characterized by the use of broad, sweeping movements that are intended to affect huge portions of the body. Sweeping motions along the length of the body are also acceptable here, as are those that sweep from side to side. The goal of these broad motions is to increase blood flow, reduce muscle tension, and create a sense of internal calm and relaxation.

• Lomi Lomi may also include stretching and joint mobilization techniques to aid in flexibility, range of motion, and the relief of joint tension. These methods often entail slow, rhythmic movements of the limbs and joints that are meant to induce a state of calm and mobility.

• Lomi Lomi practitioners may employ kneading and circular motions to release knots and stress in the body. Massage therapists may knead the muscles or provide circular pressure to the muscles using their hands, forearms, or elbows. These methods are excellent for relieving muscle tension and knots, increasing blood flow, and calming the mind.

• Healing on an energetic level is possible with the incorporation of energy work into Lomi Lomi, such as the use of intention, breathwork, and visualization. It is possible for practitioners to use their intuition and connection to the body of the recipient to detect and correct any energetic blocks or imbalances, restoring balance and fostering a state of well-being.

Lomi Lomi is a style of bodywork that may be tailored to the specific needs of both the practitioner and the person receiving the treatment. The aforementioned methods are just a sampling of the fundamental strokes and movements often utilized in Lomi Lomi; a qualified practitioner will adapt the session to the specific requirements and preferences of each individual client for an exceptional, life-altering result.

CHAPTER THREE
The Role Of Flow And Body Mechanics

Lomi Lomi relies heavily on the body's mechanics and the flow of the massage to achieve its desired effects. Body mechanics and flow are highlighted for the following reasons in Lomi Lomi:

• Maximum efficacy and efficiency in massage application are achieved through the use of correct body mechanics and flow in Lomi Lomi. Maintaining a relaxed and centered posture, employing the major muscles of the body, and providing the appropriate amount of pressure all contribute to the practitioner's ability to more precisely and efficiently administer the massage techniques. This enables for a more efficient treatment that is better able to relieve stress, ease tension, and speed recovery.

• Both the practitioner and the recipient can benefit from paying attention to their body mechanics and the flow of the exercise to maximize comfort and safety.

By avoiding unnecessary muscle and joint strain, practitioners can protect themselves from potential health problems. In addition, the receiver is more likely to relax and reap the advantages of the massage if the therapist makes an effort to ensure their comfort by using fluid, rhythmic movements and good body mechanics.

• Flow and Rhythm: Lomi Lomi relies heavily on flow and rhythm, which help to create a one-of-a-kind and profoundly soothing massage experience. Movements in Lomi Lomi are fluid and continuous, much like the rhythm of the ocean's waves, and serve to foster feelings of oneness and peace.

Using correct body mechanics and flow, the massage therapist is able to sustain a continuous stream of movements that serves to increase the massage's rhythm and flow for the benefit of the receiver.

• The energetic connection between the practitioner and the recipient is facilitated by the mechanics and flow of the practitioner's body. When two people engage in Lomi Lomi, they engage in an energetic and spiritual exchange that goes beyond a simple massage.

To attune to the recipient's energy and respond more intuitively and holistically to their needs, the practitioner must first connect with their own body, breath, and intuition through proper body mechanics and flow.

• Lomi Lomi's unique body mechanics and flow call for the practitioner to be present, mindful, and wholly immersed in the massage experience. The practitioner can then respond to the patient's requirements with complete awareness of his or her own body, breath, and energy. The practitioner's potential to provide a profoundly healing and transformational experience for the recipient is enhanced when they enter a meditative state of mind while practicing Lomi Lomi with correct body mechanics and flow.

Ultimately, the Lomi Lomi massage's efficiency, efficacy, comfort, safety, flow, rhythm, energetic connection, mindfulness, and presence are all enhanced by the practitioner's body mechanics and flow.

When performed by someone who has mastered the mechanics and flow of Lomi Lomi, the experience can be immensely healing and transformational, allowing the recipient to feel deeply relaxed, letting go of tension, and finding harmony in body, mind, and spirit.

Customs And Practices Adherent To The Lomi Lomi Tradition

Although it is a physical method, traditional Lomi Lomi massage also has spiritual and ceremonial significance in Hawaiian culture.

Many different protocols and rituals are used to show respect for the patient, make the environment sacred, and promote a more complete recovery. Some of the following customs and procedures from the Lomi Lomi tradition may be incorporated into a session:

• Traditional Lomi Lomi sessions often start with an opening ritual to set the goal, create a holy place, and invite the presence of ancestors, guides, and deities to provide blessings and protection.

This may involve reciting a prayer or mantra, lighting incense, or smudging with sacred herbs. Also, at the end of the session, a closing ceremony can be done to show appreciation, let go of any energy that were cleared or transformed, and offer closure to the whole thing.

• Before beginning a Lomi Lomi session, the practitioner may choose to conduct a ceremony to cleanse and purify the space. In order to facilitate the healing process, it may be helpful to clear the area with sacred herbs, create an altar with meaningful objects, and establish an atmosphere of calm and tranquility.

• Hawaiians frequently incorporate prayer, or "pule," into their Lomi Lomi rituals. Before or during the session, the practitioner may offer a pule to the client in order to ask for their blessings, guidance, and protection.

Hawaiian chants, invocations, or individual prayers can be used for this purpose if they are suitable for the session's goal and the person receiving the treatment.

• The setting of an intention is highly valued in Lomi Lomi. Both the healer and the person receiving treatment can benefit from working together to establish a clear intention for the session.

You can set your intention silently or out loud, and it can have any number of precise aims, such as relieving stress, calming the mind, or mending broken hearts.

• To deepen the energetic connection between the practitioner and the recipient, as well as to facilitate relaxation and presence, Lomi Lomi frequently incorporates conscious breathwork.

If the practitioner feels it would be beneficial, they could instruct the patient to slow their breathing and time it to the rhythm of the massage strokes.

• Consent and bodily consciousness are essential concepts in traditional Lomi Lomi. The provider may ask questions about the patient's general well-being, treatment choices, and any areas of particular concern.

The practitioner listens carefully to the client and adapts their techniques, pressure, and overall approach to meet the client's needs and preferences at all times.

• Traditional Lomi Lomi places a premium on the cultivation of awareness and presence. The therapist is urged to tune in intently to the recipient's body, breath, and energy, and to act accordingly. The practitioner can then tailor their care to the individual's current requirements and help bring about healing on all levels (mental, emotional, physical, and spiritual) simultaneously.

• In order to provide closure to the experience, a traditional Lomi Lomi session may include a closing ritual. Thank yous, blessings, and advice or recommendations for taking care of oneself in the days after a session are all possible ways to do this. The final ceremony is performed to show respect for the patient and the healing process, and to highlight the significance of the event.

The specific rites and protocols of Lomi Lomi may change based on the lineage, history, and philosophy of the practitioner.

CHAPTER FOUR
Different Types Of Lomi Lomi

Because of its long history and wide range of practitioners, lineages, and cultural influences, the Hawaiian massage known as Lomi Lomi has developed over time. This has led to the development of numerous subgenres of Lomi Lomi. Some well-known forms and modifications of Lomi Lomi include:

• Lomi Haa is a special kind of Lomi Lomi in which the practitioner uses his or her feet to make long, sweeping sweeps across the body.

The practitioner may apply pressure and make flowing movements with their feet and toes to generate a profound and rooted sensation. Lomi Haa has a solid reputation for being sturdy and grounded in the land.

• Lomi Haa Haa is a variant of Lomi Lomi that differs from the standard form by moving at a quicker tempo and with more intensity. A sense of velocity and flow is achieved by the use of forearms, elbows, and hands in a series of rapid and rhythmic actions. Energizing and energizing the body is a common goal of Lomi Haa Haa, which may involve stretches and joint rotations.

• Lomi Pohaku, or "Stone Massage," is a type of Hawaiian massage that makes use of heated or cooled stones. Practitioners utilize stones to exert pressure, glide, or tap along the body's energy lines and muscles. The therapeutic effects of a massage are amplified by the heat or cold from the stones, respectively.

• Long, sweeping gestures that reach from head to toe characterize this Lomi Lomi style known as Lomi Loa. The therapist may utilize their hands, forearms, and elbows to produce smooth, flowing strokes that build momentum and rapport.

Lomi Loa is revered for its calming and soothing effects, which it attributes to its caring and comforting nature.

• There is a spiritual and ceremonial component to the Temple Style of Lomi Lomi, which is informed by the teachings and practices of Hawaiian temple healers.

Invoking blessings, guidance, and healing energies may be a part of Temple Style Lomi Lomi through the use of chants, prayers, and other ritualistic aspects. Massage is more than just a relaxing experience for many people; it is also seen as a spiritual and ceremonial practice.

• Ohana Lomi Lomi is a kind of Lomi Lomi that stresses the value of ties to family and neighborhood. "Ohana" means family in Hawaiian, and Ohana Lomi Lomi is all about making you feel at home and loved. Mother-like touch techniques are sometimes used to help the receiver feel at ease, promote healing, and strengthen bonds with friends and family.

• Lomi Kuuipo is a type of Lomi Lomi that emphasizes a light, caring touch. Lomi Kuuipo, whose name comes from the Hawaiian word for "sweetheart," places an emphasis on providing a kind and affectionate massage.

It is characterized by slow, smooth, flowing motions that evoke feelings of love and caring; these help with stress reduction, emotional healing, and bonding.

It is worth noting that there may be some overlap between the numerous Lomi Lomi styles and variations, and that individual practitioners may draw from a variety of sources when developing their own distinctive approach.

Finding a practitioner with whom you have a good rapport and communicating openly are crucial for having a positive and stress-free encounter.

Lomi Lomi And The Brain, Body, And Soul

Traditional Hawaiian massage, or Lomi Lomi, takes a holistic perspective by attending to the whole person, including the mind, body, and spirit.

It is a form of massage that takes into account the full person, not just their physical needs, and so works on their mental, emotional, and spiritual well-being as well. Lomi Lomi's philosophy and beliefs, as well as the massage's strokes, rituals, and emphasis on the mind-body connection, are inextricably intertwined.

• Lomi Lomi practitioners understand the significance of mental health to overall health. The massage therapist keeps in mind the client's emotional state and strives to cultivate an atmosphere of serenity and safety in order to alleviate stress and anxiety. Lomi Lomi strokes are characterized by rhythmic, flowing movements that aim to calm the mind and put the recipient into a state of deep relaxation.

• Lomi Lomi is primarily concerned with the physical body, and its techniques and strokes are intended to work on the body's muscles, tissues, and energy channels.

Long, flowing strokes, as well as the practitioner's forearms, elbows, and other body parts, are used to reduce muscle tension, increase blood flow, and facilitate relaxation and healing.

• Soul or Spirit: Lomi Lomi places great value on the well-being of a person's spirit or soul. Some practitioners may add spiritual aspects to the massage, such as chants, prayers, or blessings, and the work is done with intention and regard.

The purpose of a Lomi Lomi session is to revitalize the recipient's energy and foster feelings of peace and oneness with the universe.

Lomi Lomi emphasizes a connection between the recipient's mind, body, and spirit that lasts long after the massage is over.

Lomi Lomi promotes a comprehensive view of health by emphasizing the importance of self-care, self-awareness, and mindfulness. As a ceremonial practice, giving and receiving a massage is thought to break down emotional barriers, inspire introspection, and facilitate growth and change.

Overall, Lomi Lomi acknowledges the interconnectedness and interdependence of the mind, body, and spirit, and that it is necessary to address all areas of a person's being to achieve optimal health and well-being. It promotes wellness on all levels, from the physical to the emotional.

CHAPTER FIVE
Theories Of Hawaiian Health And Wholeness

Well-being and completeness are notions that have profound cultural and spiritual roots in Hawaii.

Hawaiian health and wellness traditions recognize the importance of mind, body, spirit, and environment in obtaining complete health and happiness.

Some of the most fundamental tenets of Hawaiian views on health and completeness are:

• The Hawaiian idea of pono entails
a pursuit of equilibrium, harmony,
and morality. It entails acting in
harmony with one's actual self and
the laws of nature.

When discussing health and
wellness, pono stresses the necessity
of a holistic approach that takes into
account one's physical, mental,
emotional, and spiritual states. Self-
care, good relationships,
environmental stewardship, and
acting in accordance with one's core
values and principles all figure
prominently.

• In Hawaiian culture, "Aloha" is more than a simple welcome or farewell expression. It is a deep idea that includes all kinds of caring and bonding. Aloha, when applied to health, stresses the significance of loving oneself, one's fellow humans, and the planet. Kindness, respect, and empathy are essential components, as is an awareness of the interdependence of all forms of life.

• Ohana: Ohana is the Hawaiian idea of family, which includes not only biological relatives but also friends and extended acquaintances.

Ohana is a Hawaiian concept that refers to the value of family, friends, and community in maintaining health and happiness. It acknowledges that people are social creatures who do best in communities where they have friends and family to lean on.

• Mana is a Hawaiian term that refers to a person's life force or their spiritual essence. It is the vital force that animates everything and links the natural world together.

Mana, in the context of health, stresses the value of developing one's spirituality. Meditation, prayer, and spending time in nature are all part of this approach, which aims to promote and sustain a healthy spiritual life.

• The Hawaiian idea of 'lama refers to the duty of caretaking and responsibility. It stresses the significance of caring for oneself, one's community, and one's natural surroundings.

Wellness as it pertains to mlama entails not just caring for others and the environment, but also taking care of oneself via self-care, self-compassion, and self-awareness. It acknowledges that one's own happiness depends on the happiness of others and the earth.

These are only a few of the pillars around which Hawaiian ideas of health and completeness are built. Lomi Lomi massage and other traditional Hawaiian techniques utilize these ideas to foster health on all levels: mental, physical, spiritual, and environmental.

Living in accordance with these ideas and principles can help you feel more at peace and whole, which in turn improves your health and well-being.

Lomi Lomi's Energical Precepts

Since Lomi Lomi is a traditional Hawaiian massage, it naturally combines energy principles thought to play a significant role in health and healing.

Hawaiian belief in the body's energy and spiritual nature is the basis for these energetic concepts. Lomi Lomi's energizing concepts consist of:

• The Hawaiian notion of mana, often known as life force or spiritual energy, permeates all forms of life.

The goal of a Lomi Lomi practitioner is to increase the mana of the person receiving the treatment as well as the person administering it. To facilitate healing, the practitioner channels their own mana, as well as that of the surrounding landscape and their ancestors.

• In Hawaiian culture, the word "aloha" is more than just a greeting; it also carries a potent dynamic idea. It is a vital force that is thought to run all throughout the body, and it is associated with feelings of love, compassion, and connection.

The therapist infuse the massage with aloha (love, respect, and compassion) in Lomi Lomi. It is considered that this kind of loving presence can help with healing and generate a balanced flow of energy.

• Movement and Flow: Lomi Lomi massage uses lengthy, flowing strokes with a steady rhythm to evoke feelings of motion and flow.

There is a belief that these sweeping strokes can assist clear stagnant energy, increase mana flow, and relieve stress on a physical and emotional level. The practitioner moves with dance-like fluidity and grace, using their body to create a unified and harmonious energetic field for the recipient.

• During a Lomi Lomi massage, the therapist is urged to rely on his or her intuition and to be fully present. They let their intuition and strong connection to the energy of the recipient to direct their motions and approaches.

This intuitive method allows the practitioner to tailor the healing process to the specific needs of the patient on the physical, mental, emotional, and spiritual planes.

• Lomi Lomi is often regarded as a spiritual and ceremonial rite in

Hawaiian society. Rituals, prayers, and blessings are sometimes incorporated into traditional Lomi Lomi to pay respect to the receiver, the ancestors, and the natural world.

These spiritual aids are thought to raise the massage's energetic vibration, forging a closer bond with the divine and fostering a sense of harmony and balance.

Lomi Lomi massage is based on these and other energetic principles. Mana, aloha, flow, intuition, and sacredness are all emphasized as crucial to the practice of Lomi Lomi, as is the connectivity of mind, body, spirit, and environment.

Practitioners of Lomi Lomi attempt to promote the recipient's overall balance, harmony, and well-being by incorporating these energetic principles into their work.

CHAPTER SIX
The Physical, Emotional, And Mental Benefits Of Lomi Lomi

Lomi Lomi is a form of holistic and therapeutic massage that has been shown to have positive effects on a person's physical health, as well as their mental and emotional well-being.

The concepts of Hawaiian medicine, which are the basis for these advantages, place an emphasis on the connectivity of body, mind, and spirit and the development of holistic health. The following are some of the therapeutic advantages of Lomi Lomi:

• Lomi Lomi is a form of massage that focuses on relieving physical stress and tension through the use of long, gliding strokes, stretches, and joint rotations. The massage's soft yet firm pressure helps ease muscle soreness, stiffness, and pain while also promoting a state of deep physical relaxation.

• Because of its emphasis on stretching and joint mobilization, Lomi Lomi can be helpful for persons with mobility issues or stiffness in certain parts of the body to increase their overall flexibility and range of motion.

• Lomi Lomi massage is thought to stimulate the lymphatic system, which is responsible for the evacuation of toxins from the body, leading to detoxification and enhanced immunity. Lomi Lomi's fluid motions and rhythmic strokes may aid lymphatic drainage, which in turn may aid in detoxification and immune system support.

• Lomi Lomi is well-known for its calming and nurturing effects, which make it useful for relieving stress, anxiety, and tension. The practitioner's caring presence, together with the soothing music and gentle motions, can help the client feel at ease and enhance emotional health.

• Lomi Lomi is thought to increase mental clarity and attention by helping to quiet the mind. Because of the profound level of relaxation it induces, getting a massage can be a great way to clear your head, calm your nerves, and focus your thoughts.

• Lomi Lomi promotes introspection and an enhanced connection between the body and the mind. The combination of the practitioner's intuitive touch with the flowing movements can help the receiver develop a stronger sense of connection and awareness between their mind and body.

• The energetic principles of Lomi Lomi, including mana, aloha, flow, and sacredness, are said to create energetic balance and alignment. Lomi Lomi is thought to improve a person's health and vitality by breaking up energy blocks, increasing the flow of mana, and rebalancing the recipient's energy.

• Lomi Lomi has been defined as a very caring and nourishing experience for the whole person, including the mind and spirit.

The recipient is able to unwind, let go, and receive care and support in a sacred and safe environment brought about by the practitioner's smooth strokes, warm presence, and the sanctity of the practice.

People feel that receiving Lomi Lomi on all levels—physical, mental, and emotional—can help them heal more completely. Lomi Lomi should only be received from a skilled and experienced practitioner to avoid any unwanted side effects and to maximize any potential benefits.

Setting Intentions And Creating A Sacred Space In Lomi Lomi

The holistic and spiritual quality of Lomi Lomi massage is enhanced by the creation of a sacred place and the setting of intention. Lomi Lomi is typically viewed as a sacred ceremony that honors the recipient's body, mind, and spirit because of its association with the Hawaiian concept of sacredness, or kapu. Key elements of Lomi Lomi sacred space creation and intention setting include:

• Lomi Lomi should be practiced in a location that is both physically and energetically clear. A healing environment is one that allows one to feel relaxed and at peace. Achieving this can be as simple as setting the mood with the right lighting, music, aromatherapy, and furniture. Symbolic items like flowers, crystals, and other holy objects may be used by some practitioners to elevate a room to a sacred one.

• Some Lomi Lomi practitioners will undertake a clearing ritual to cleanse the space of any negative or sluggish energy before beginning a session.

One method is to smudge the area with sage or another purifying herb, ring bells or chimes, or recite prayers or chants.

• The practice of Lomi Lomi relies heavily on the setting of an intention. A session's intention can be anything from a specific aim or outcome to a more general intention for healing, relaxation, or balance, and it can be set by both the practitioner and the recipient. Having a clear aim in mind for the session helps the practitioner and the recipient channel their energy in the same direction.

• Touch in Lomi Lomi is utilized for sacred purposes such as bonding, communicating, and healing. The therapist approaches the patient with awe and care, touching them with only the best intentions. The person being touched should be receptive, letting go of any resistance to the healing power of touch.

• Mindful Presence: During a Lomi Lomi session, both the practitioner and the recipient are asked to focus their attention on the here and now and let go of any outside concerns or distractions. The practitioner and the patient can form a closer bond through mindful presence, which improves the quality of care provided.

• Lomi Lomi is commonly connected with the spirituality and connection to nature that is so central to Hawaiian culture. Some practitioners may add natural oils, flowers, or other plant-based items to further emphasize the feeling of oneness with nature. The practitioners may also create a sacred space by praying, chanting, or engaging in other spiritual acts during the session.

• Spirit of Aloha (Love, Compassion, and Respect) and

Gratitude: Two fundamental ideas in Lomi Lomi are gratitude and the spirit of aloha. It is important for both the healer and the healed to maintain an attitude of appreciation toward the body, mind, and spirit, as well as the healer, the ancestors, and the healing process as a whole. The aloha mindset fosters an environment of love and harmony, which aids in the recovery process.

When giving a Lomi Lomi massage, it is important to create a sacred place and set an intention so that the receiver can relax and enjoy the experience. It adds to the Lomi Lomi massage's profound healing and transformative capabilities and contributes to the practice's entire holistic and spiritual character.

CHAPTER SEVEN
Hawaiian Medicine: A History Of Herbal Treatments

The cultural and spiritual foundations of traditional Hawaiian healing are rock solid. The mind, emotions, and soul are all considered in these methods of healing in addition to the physical body.

In addition to Lomi Lomi massage, the following traditional Hawaiian therapeutic procedures and herbal medicines are often employed:

• Ho'oponopono is a traditional Hawaiian practice of forgiveness and reconciliation that seeks to mend fences and bring people back together after they have been at odds.

It is thought to have far-reaching effects on one's physical, mental, and emotional well-being, and it entails a process of serious self-reflection, confession, and forgiveness.

• Hawaiians have a long history of using herbal treatments derived from plants, known as La'au Lapa'au. The Hawaiian Islands are home to a wide variety of medicinal plants, and the traditional use of these plants for therapeutic purposes goes back hundreds of years in Hawaiian culture. Herbal medicines are utilized for a variety of illnesses, both medical and mental/emotional/spiritual.

• Traditional Hawaiian Lomi Lomi is known as Lomi Lomi Pa'a, and it includes chanting, prayer, and energy work in addition to the physical techniques used in modern Lomi Lomi. This ceremonial and spiritual form of Lomi Lomi works to bring the body, mind, and spirit back into harmony.

• Hawaiians traditionally worship and invoke deities via a ritual called pule. It is a way to get in touch with God and ask for help, safety, and favor. Pule is commonly used to establish a holy place and set healing intentions alongside other healing techniques like Lomi Lomi.

- A traditional Hawaiian herbal treatment, 'Awa (or kava) is utilized for its sedative and tranquilizing qualities. The calming effects of 'awa make it a popular remedy for insomnia and other sleep disturbances. Typically, the 'awa plant's roots are fermented into an alcoholic beverage.

- Traditional Hawaiian medicine makes use of a fruit called noni for its purported health benefits. Noni is utilized for a variety of diseases, including pain relief, wound healing, and immune support, due to its antioxidant, anti-inflammatory, and immune-boosting characteristics.

• Limu, or seaweed, is widely utilized in traditional Hawaiian medicine due to its nutritive and therapeutic qualities. Limu is known for its ability to reduce inflammation, eliminate toxins, and strengthen the immune system because of its abundance of beneficial vitamins, minerals, and antioxidants. It can be eaten or applied topically to treat skin problems.

Some of the traditional Hawaiian therapeutic procedures and herbal medicines that accompany a Lomi Lomi massage session include the following. Hawaiians have long believed in the holistic and interconnected nature of health and healing, and these traditions are a reflection of that view. These facets of traditional Hawaiian therapy complement the Lomi Lomi massage's focus on the full person, including the body, mind, and soul.

How To Give A Lomi Lomi Massage: A Step-By-Step Breakdown

Learning the techniques and concepts of Lomi Lomi massage takes time and dedication. Here is a high-level breakdown of how to provide a Lomi Lomi massage:

• Beginning with an intention for the massage and establishing a sacred space is the first step.

Candlelight, gentle music, and aromatic essential oils are all possible ways to achieve this state of mind. Choose a goal for the massage, such as healing, renewal, or just relaxation, and encourage the client to do the same.

• Second, get the client ready by walking them to the massage table and talking to them about what to expect from the session, such as the massage therapist's usage of forearms and elbows, and whether or not hot stones or other instruments will be used.

Get the client's approval and answer their queries before proceeding. Inquire about the patient's health background, the nature of the problem(s) they wish to treat, and their tolerance for physical contact.

• Third, commence the massage with a prayer and pule, or invocation, as is customary in Hawaiian culture. This creates a holy environment for healing, strengthens the connection with the client's spirit, and establishes the intention for the session.

• Fourth, grease up your hands and arms with heated oil, and start massaging with smooth, rhythmic strokes. Make long, sweeping motions with your arms and hands, like the waves on the ocean.

Make use of your body weight and body mechanics to move with ease and grace. Adjust the amount of pressure and speed to suit the individual. When necessary, use circular motions, kneading, and stretching.

• Fifth, go with the flow and trust your instincts; lomi lomi massage has been likened to a dance or a swaying beat. Adjust your methods and pressure based on the client's feedback and physical sensations. Keep your hands, forearms, and elbows moving in unison as you glide and sweep over your client's muscles to induce a state of calm and balance.

• Sixth, use stretching and joint mobilization techniques Stretching and joint mobilization are common components of Lomi Lomi massage, serving to alleviate muscle tension and increase range of motion. Stretch your muscles and joints gently to increase range of motion and blood flow. When stretching a client, it is important to make sure they are feeling good about it and not in any pain.

• Seventh, if desired, hot stones or other instruments are used, such as bamboo sticks or shells, to improve the massage sensation during a Lomi Lomi session. The therapeutic effects of massage are enhanced when these tools are employed to impart localized heat, pressure, or sensory stimulation. Always consult the client about their level of comfort and sensitivity before utilizing hot stones or other equipment.

• Finish the massage with a closing ritual, such as a prayer, pule, or other traditional Hawaiian practice, as described in Step 8. Finish the massage by making sure the client is relaxed and at ease with some long, sweeping strokes.

•Give Clients Advice on How to Take Care of Themselves After the Massage Recommend that the customer consume plenty of water, rest, and avoid strenuous activity for a while.

Give advice on how to take care of oneself outside of the massage, such as stretches, meditation, or other self-help techniques. Remind the client to pay attention to how they feel

CHAPTER EIGHT
Client Relaxation, Proper Body Positioning, And Draping

In order to provide a safe, professional, and enjoyable Lomi Lomi massage session for the client, proper body alignment, draping, and client comfort are essential. The following are some suggestions:

• Client Body Positioning: Place the client in a relaxed and comfortable position on the massage table. Lomi Lomi massage is characterized by long, sweeping strokes, therefore the practitioner needs plenty of room to maneuver around the table. The practitioner and patient can agree on whether the patient should lie face up or face down.

• Clients' privacy and comfort should be protected with proper draping techniques used during the massage. Cover the client with a sheet, towel, or sarong, and only expose the area being operated on. Adjust the drapes as needed during the session to ensure that the client is completely at ease.

• To guarantee the client's comfort throughout the massage, it is important to check in with them at regular intervals. Inquire as to the level of pressure, temperature, and any other pain they may be feeling.

Make adjustments to your approach and level of pressure based on their comments and wishes. Make sure the client is warm and comfortable by using cushions or bolsters to support their body and joints.

• In Lomi Lomi massage, communication is essential. It is important to make sure the client feels safe to share their thoughts and feelings during the session.

Pay attention to the comments they have, and modify your methods as needed. Make sure the client is aware of the massage's progression, any adjustments to the pressure, and the last ritual to keep them relaxed and at ease.

• Maintain a professional demeanor and treat the customer with the utmost respect at all times.

Keep your distance and protect their anonymity and privacy. Facilitate the client's ability to unwind, let go, and experience the therapeutic effects of Lomi Lomi massage by providing a calm, accepting environment.

Keep in mind that the individual Lomi Lomi massage method being done, as well as local restrictions and requirements, may necessitate certain adjustments to body alignment, draping, and client comfort. Maintain the greatest level of professionalism at all times and put the needs of the client first at all times.

Problems And Obstacles In Lomi-Lomi And How To Fix Them

Practitioners of Lomi Lomi may face similar difficulties and obstacles to those encountered by those learning other types of massage. Some typical difficulties and troubles in Lomi Lomi, along with solutions, are as follows:

• The use of lengthy, flowing strokes and body motions is characteristic of Lomi Lomi, which can be physically taxing for the practitioner.

Careful attention to body mechanics, alignment, and the avoidance of unnecessary stress and strain should be the focus of any practitioner. Self-care routines like stretching, exercise, and bodywork can alleviate stress and tension in the body.

• Practitioner fatigue: Lomi Lomi sessions can last a long time and be strenuous on the body. Practitioners should pace themselves, drink plenty of water, and avoid getting too hungry or too tired during sessions.

To avoid burnout and keep themselves healthy, professionals should get plenty of sleep and practice self-care.

• Lomi Lomi's integrative nature and emphasis on the link between the mind, body, and spirit have been linked to the experience of emotional release in certain individuals.

The practitioner should be able to "hold space" for the client when they experience difficult feelings like sadness, grief, or rage. Provide necessary support and advice while responding with empathy, compassion, and nonjudgment.

• The practice of Lomi Lomi should be approached with cultural awareness and respect, as it has its origins in Hawaiian tradition.

Practitioners should learn about the historical context and accepted practices of Lomi Lomi from experienced practitioners or Hawaiian elders. Avoid distorting or appropriating Lomi Lomi and show respect for its historical and cultural roots to ensure its survival.

• Client Relaxation: Relaxation is a top priority for a successful Lomi Lomi session. Some customers can feel uneasy with all the touching and bending and slathering with oil.

Practitioners should always get clients' informed consent, explain any unusual procedures or clothing changes ahead of time, and make sure they are comfortable at all times during the session. Make any necessary adjustments to the client's pressure, positioning, and drape to ensure their safety and comfort.

• Limits and Ethics: As with any type of massage, it is crucial to uphold professional limits and ethical standards when practicing Lomi Lomi.

Professionals owe it to their patients and clients to set limits on their interactions with them, protect their privacy, and act ethically at all times. All elements of your Lomi

Lomi practice should be conducted with the utmost professionalism, integrity, and ethics.

Practitioners of Lomi Lomi can better ensure their customers' safety, comfort, and well-being during sessions by keeping in mind these frequently encountered obstacles.

Lomi Lomi massage is beneficial to the health of both the practitioner and the client, but only if the therapist maintains a high level of competence through ongoing training, self-care, and adherence to professional norms and ethics.

CHAPTER NINE

How To Use Lomi Lomi In Your Massage Therapy Business

Adding the comprehensive and one-of-a-kind Lomi Lomi massage technique to your practice can be quite satisfying. If you are interested in incorporating Lomi Lomi into your massage therapy, here are some things to think about:

• Lomi Lomi is a unique style of massage with its own set of rules and traditions, thus it is important to learn how to do it correctly. If you want to learn Lomi Lomi properly, you need to find a practitioner or teacher with experience in the field. Learn the fundamentals, advanced techniques, cultural relevance, and ethical considerations of Lomi Lomi by enrolling in a respected training program.

• Get to know the underlying principles of Lomi Lomi, such as the importance of purpose setting and the energy principles at play, and the value of the mind-body link. With this knowledge, you will be better equipped to incorporate the distinctive elements of Lomi Lomi into your practice and offer a more comprehensive service to your customers.

• One of the basic tenets of Lomi Lomi is the establishment of a sacred space. Create an atmosphere befitting the spiritual significance of massage. Create a tranquil and relaxing atmosphere with the help of

Hawaiian-themed furnishings, low lighting, soothing music, and natural materials like plants, stones, and shells.

• Before beginning each Lomi Lomi session, it is helpful to establish your intentions for the session.

Connecting with the client's body, mind, and spirit in the present moment is central to the practice of Lomi Lomi. Enhance the mind-body connection through Lomi Lomi by including breathwork, meditation, and mindful touch.

• Lomi Lomi strokes and methods should be incorporated into your sessions. These include lengthy, flowing strokes, joint rotations, and stretches. Create a rhythm and flow that resembles the ocean waves with your forearms, palms, and fingers; this is a crucial part of Lomi Lomi.

• Please take into account the cultural context in which Lomi Lomi is being performed. Lomi Lomi has a rich cultural history that should be respected and honored. Make sure you are practicing Lomi Lomi with cultural sensitivity and respect by learning about its history, customs, and norms.

• Client Communication: Be sure to keep your clients in the loop regarding your Lomi Lomi session's goals, draping, and other specifics. Clients should give their informed permission once all of their questions and worries have been addressed. In order to make your customers feel at ease during the session, it is important to brief them on the specifics of Lomi Lomi and what they can expect.

• Learn as much as you can as often as you can; Lomi Lomi is a vast and complex field, and you need to keep learning if you want to master it. Keep up with the state-of-the-art in

Lomi Lomi studies, methods, and customs. To deepen your knowledge of Lomi Lomi and increase your skill level, it is recommended that you participate in workshops, seminars, and trainings.

• Lomi Lomi can be taxing on the body and the spirit, so it is necessary for practitioners to make time for rest and rejuvenation.

Take care of yourself by engaging in self-care practices like stretching, exercise, meditation, and frequent bodywork to avoid burnout and keep your energy up.

If you want to include Lomi Lomi into your massage practice, you need to learn everything you can about its history, philosophy, principles, and practices.

Offering a genuinely therapeutic and culturally sensitive approach to massage is possible when you incorporate the distinctive characteristics of Lomi Lomi into your practice and provide a comprehensive experience for your clients.

Conclusion

The ancient Hawaiian art of Lomi Lomi massage takes a multifaceted, holistic approach by focusing on the relationship between body, mind, and spirit.

Lomi Lomi is a healing and enlightening experience for the practitioner and the client thanks to its rich cultural past, distinctive techniques, and philosophical ideas.

The benefits of Lomi Lomi on physical, mental, and emotional levels, as well as its underlying concepts and philosophy, historical and cultural context, basic techniques and strokes, energetic principles, traditional rites and protocols, are all discussed in this guide.

Body mechanics, flow, intention setting, and the creation of a holy place have also been covered as they pertain to Lomi Lomi.

To successfully incorporate Lomi Lomi into your massage practice, you must first acquire the necessary training, cultural knowledge, mindfulness, and ongoing education.

Self-care, open communication with clients, and honoring Lomi Lomi's traditions and regulations are all essential to becoming a successful practitioner.

Including Lomi Lomi in your massage therapy sessions is a great way to stand apart from the crowd, while also paying tribute to the rich cultural history of this traditional Hawaiian method of healing. Lomi Lomi may be a life-changing experience for both you and your customers, regardless of whether you are an experienced massage therapist or just starting out.

THE END

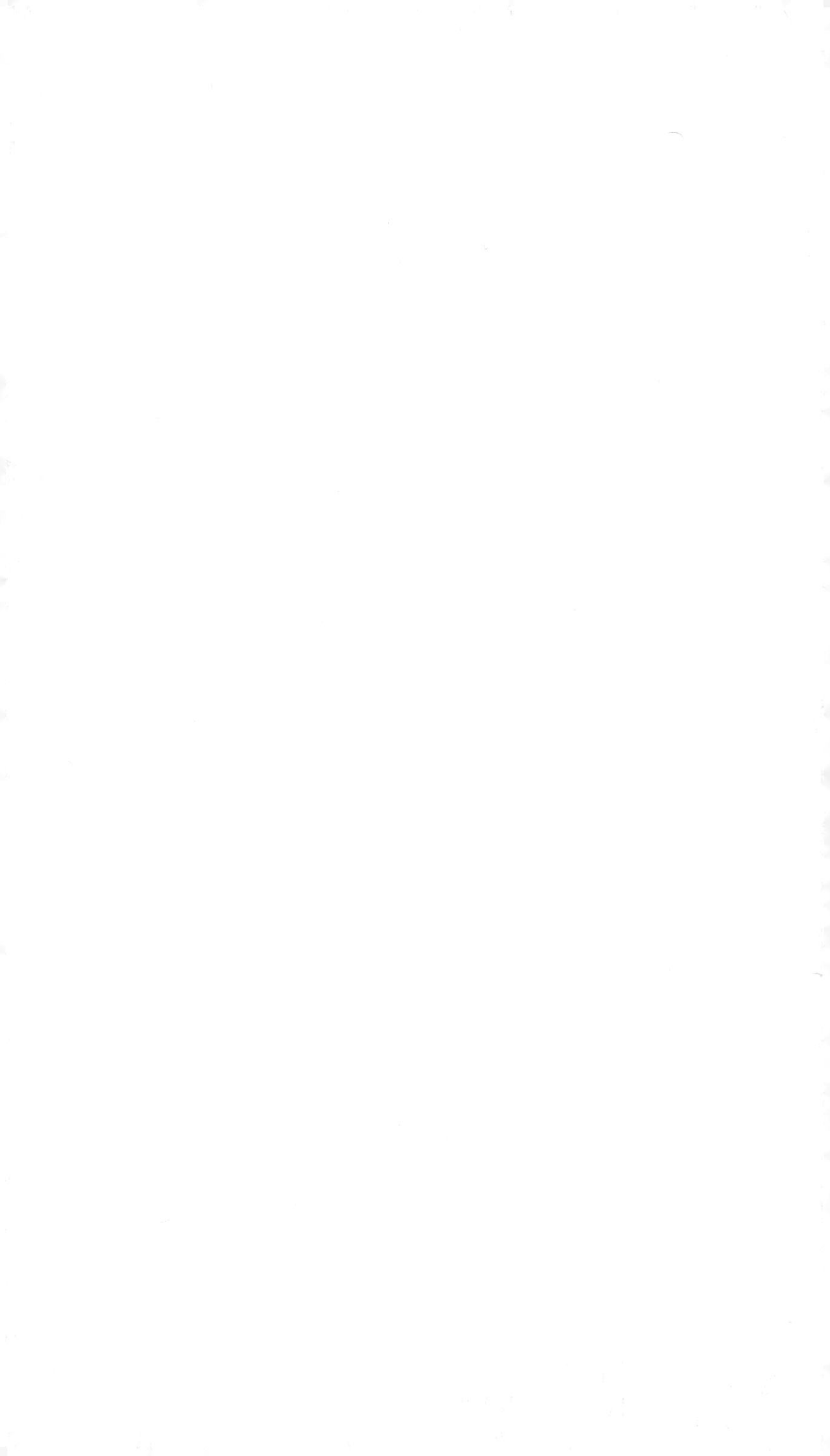